BUTLER'S
DMT
FIELD GUIDE

*A Brief History, Step-by-Step Recipes,
and Personal Experiences From a DMT
Saturated Consciousness*

ADAM D. BUTLER

First Stillwater River Publications Edition.

ISBN: 978-1-960505-05-7

1 2 3 4 5 6 7 8 9 10
Written by Adam D. Butler.
Cover & interior book design by Matthew St. Jean.
Published by Stillwater River Publications, Pawtucket, RI, USA.

Names: Butler, Adam D., author.
Title: Butler's DMT field guide : a brief history, step-by-step recipes, and personal experiences from a DMT saturated consciousness / Adam D. Butler.
Description: First Stillwater River Publications edition. | Pawtucket, RI, USA : Stillwater River Publications, [2023]
Identifiers: ISBN: 978-1-960505-05-7 (paperback)
Subjects: LCSH: Butler, Adam D.--Mental health. | Dimethyltryptamine--Therapeutic use--Handbooks, manuals, etc. | Dimethyltryptamine--Physiological effect--Handbooks, manuals, etc. | Hallucinogenic drugs--Therapeutic use--Handbooks, manuals, etc. | Hallucinogenic drugs--Physiological effect--Handbooks, manuals, etc. | LCGFT: Handbooks and manuals.
Classification: LCC: RM666.D564 B88 2023 | DDC: 615.7883--dc23

Disclaimer

The ideas, recipes, and experiences expressed in this book are from my personal exploration of dimethyltryptamine. I am not a medical doctor, nor am I giving medical advice. Laws are different depending on what country you live in; please do not do anything that is unlawful or unsafe. There are chemicals and processes outlined in this book that can be extremely dangerous, and can cause serious bodily harm if proper precautions are not followed. The ingredients used in the DMT brew have been reported to have adverse interactions with several types of prescription medications related to MAOIs (monoamine oxidase inhibitors), and you should consult your doctor if you have any concerns. Once you use DMT, your perception of the external world, as well as your self-awareness, will forever be altered. You will *not* be able go back to the old way of "seeing" things. Have an open mind, and enjoy the incredible experience, but please be careful and responsible. Do your own research, ask questions, and make sure you have the proper intentions during all stages of your journey.

Contents

Changing Gears
Custom metal art by Nick Marshall

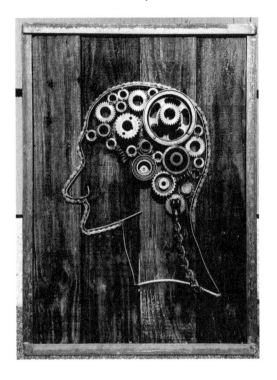

Changing Gears is the title of this compelling and beautiful custom piece of art by my friend Nick Marshall, and it is the perfect visual and conceptual metaphor for what DMT can do to one's thought process and direction of life. We all have our own issues and mental road blocks, and whether you need to up shift, down shift, go into park, or change course and go into reverse, I hope the words in the following pages will help enlighten your journey.

CHAPTER 1

Who the Fuck Am I?

"Who the fuck am i?" to anyone who has ever looked into the sky and desperately pleaded with the Universe to give some insight into this query, the words in this book will hopefully provide some guidance. The question posed in this chapter title, albeit considered vulgar by some, is just one of many existential and eternal questions that DMT will help the human species come closer to answering. It is a question I have asked myself many times, and is one I recommend you ask yourself prior to using DMT.

Before we delve deep into philosophical dialogue, and more importantly before you trust me enough to offer advice on experimenting with one of the strongest psychedelic drugs known to science, it is important for the reader to know who I am. Who *is* the author of this book, and why should you continue to read it? Why should its content be considered worthy of your time, as well as be added to the lexicon and database of information on this particular topic? If you decide to explore the benefits of DMT, your perception of the physical and spiritual world around you will be dramatically changed. You will undoubtedly become a different person. For me to accurately describe who I am, or more importantly why you should give my words any value or weight, I must describe my life in terms of "before DMT," and "after DMT."

My forty-plus years of life on this planet before DMT read like a Greek tragedy. For the sake of brevity, and to avoid sounding conceited or self-absorbed, the next paragraph is purposely void of many details, and written simply to give a brief overview of my life prior to dimethyltryptamine.

It starts off poetically beautiful, and then goes gruesomely horrible. I was the blue-eyed golden child that could do no wrong, and who was raised with a silver spoon in his mouth. My entire life I have had the encouragement and support of an amazing cast of family, friends, teachers, and mentors. Every physical and material need was either generously handed to me, or was abnormally easy for me to personally obtain. Each spontaneous desire, quickly satiated. All of my dreams were magically realized. I breezed through high school and college with high grades, great memories, and every goal achieved. I received scholarships, grants, and accolades. I had the pleasure to attend the University of Rhode Island and absorb the intellectual and spiritual wisdom of some of the world's most learned minds. I was taken under the wings of two of the top scientists in the field of entomology, who not only shared my passion and complete awe of the insect world, but also buzzed with the innate calling to help humankind by applying their knowledge to lessen the pain and suffering of others. I have been exposed to, and have read, thousands and thousands of books, and have been able to internalize the thoughts of some of the most profound thinkers of the world, spanning from the time of the spoken word to the present. I have made love to some of the most beautiful women on the planet, owned my dream homes, cars, and toys, etc. I have experienced financial abundance, expressed myself artistically, traveled the world, owned my own businesses, have always been extremely lucky, healthy, blessed...blah blah.... Fucking blah.

Those "positive" things were mentioned in the prior paragraph to put this one into proper perspective. Everything in my personal world burned to the ground over the course of the last two and a half years. Even worse, I brought a bunch of loved ones down with me. I had two heart-crushing relationship breakups, left two dream jobs because of my mental illness, had emergency hemorrhoid surgery while awake, sold all my properties and became homeless (moved back in with my parents after previously owning fifteen houses), almost killed an innocent man (literally was going to end someone's life over

$900), sold off my retirement savings and drained all my bank accounts, maxed out my credit cards to fund a year of living on the road....

To wrap a nice bow around this lovely picture...I had a complete mental breakdown and went out into the desert to kill myself by a combination of drugs, speed, knives, and self-pity. I was *now* the red-eyed, suicidal maniac who had nothing except a stomach full of snot and tears, a blade piercing his throat, and veins bulging on his temples. I had submitted. I had tapped out. I was done wanting to exist. *I closed my eyes to die.*

My brain could not reconcile my internal conflicts, nor alleviate my mental pain. I possessed every possible advantage any person could ever ask for, and then some. There was not one factor in the outside world or part of my physical body or environment I would change, but my mental state was a complete and utter disaster. Every well-intentioned loved one, friend, or doctor immediately pleaded with me to ingest some pill that would drug me up beyond recognition. Basically, everyone wanted to dull my senses and stop me from expressing my thoughts and feelings in an honest and personal way. With the sincerest of intentions, they all wanted to take my unique light and darken it, because that was the easy, socially accepted way of dealing with someone like myself. Someone who was clearly "crazy."

Simply turning down the volume of my craziness was not an option in my opinion. I wanted to explore and understand the source of my problems, not just sweep them under the rug; and besides, my unique mental abilities are what allowed me to excel in life, and what has set me apart from the mundane and mediocre. My craziness is what made me special; however, I needed to understand why my brain was having such a hard time dealing with everyday issues like calm communication in my close relationships, having a positive self-image and self-esteem, and knowing how to quiet my mind at the end of the day.

I was painfully aware that I have had it better off than a huge percentage of the world's population, and this was certainly not making it any easier for me to process my perceived inadequacies. There was absolutely no reason for me to be bitching about anything, let alone ready to give up on life because it was too hard. "What a fucking Sally!" I had to find the keys to unlock my mental blocks. It was honestly a matter of life and death, and I knew that some doctor who sees a dozen patients a day, and gives everyone the same cocktail of prescription pills, was NOT the holder of those keys.

I had to balance my mental, physical, and spiritual ledgers. I needed to get the hell out of my own way. This was a process and journey I had to complete myself. There weren't going to be any shortcuts, and I knew I could not depend on someone else to understand, let alone "fix" my deepest and darkest issues. The sick feeling in my stomach confirmed I had only one path, and one option.

I had to explore every putrid and dank corner and nook of my ego and psyche. I had to scrape out and remove all the bullshit and self-sabotage that had accumulated over my adult life. I needed to locate and get rid of the plaque that was not only preventing my unique light from shining from within, but also blocked me from absorbing the healing light from the universal field.

DMT handed me the keys...*and* the map, *and* a flashlight, *and* a personally guided tour of the inner workings of my consciousness. DMT saved my life! It is for *that* reason that I feel compelled to share my research and experiences. It is not with any intention of glorifying DMT, or making it mainstream, but with a genuine desire to potentially help just one person who may have travelled to the same rancid recesses of their mind and soul that I did. I am hoping to help move the discussion forward on dimethyltryptamine, and to increase the understanding of our physiological relationship to it. My experiences, both horrifically dark and magically wonderful, will hopefully give some comfort to the parents, loved ones, and medical professionals that are desperately trying to ease the pain of that tortured someone they are attempting to console.

Dimethyltryptamine has been the subject of some fantastic and incredibly thorough academic research and clinical studies; there is, however, not much available information relating to practical, non-laboratory use of this molecule. I could not find a comprehensive guide that I trusted to walk me through a DMT session from beginning to end. There was no literature or YouTube video that explained everything from "soup to nuts," or in my case, explained everything from "DMT brew to going nuts." With my scientific background, I could understand and appreciate not only the data that was collected, but also the limitations that were dutifully imposed on the "professional" research. With my prior experience using psychedelic drugs, and my batshit crazy way of thinking, I could also understand and appreciate the stories of the volunteers, shamans, and luminaries that beautifully articulated their DMT sessions and epiphanies. The more I became familiar with DMT, the more I felt compelled to share what I had found in my research, as well as what I had experienced during my personal sessions.

Butler's DMT Field Guide is intended to be a helpful introduction to anyone who may be interested in dimethyltryptamine. I was seeking a book similar to this when I was doing my research into DMT, and I approached writing it from that perspective. My intent is to provide practical and potentially novel insight to assist my fellow psychonauts to safely take off and land, and at the same time *not* piss off the scientists and medical professionals that I admire and respect. My goal is to help bridge the gap between what has been uncovered from the structured scientific and medical studies, and the knowledge that has been gleaned from "real world" DMT experiences of the bold people who have taken the leap into the boundless unknown.

This book provides recipes that I have used to make both DMT brew and DMT crystals, discusses methods of consumption and dosing guidelines, and shares my personal experiences to hopefully help make a DMT newcomer's journey as smooth and enlightening as possible. It is a genuine, and heartfelt desire, that the following pages will help shed some light on what in my experience has been a true Miracle Molecule. A molecule that helped save my life.

CHAPTER 2

DMT: The Miracle Molecule

Dr. RICK STRASSMAN, A MEDICALLY TRAINED PROFES-sional and one of the leading scientific minds who has researched dimethyltryptamine, used the term "Spirit Molecule" in his eye-opening and groundbreaking book *DMT, The Spirit Molecule: A Doctor's Revolutionary Research into the Biology of Near-Death and Mystical Experiences.* Coining DMT as the "Spirit" molecule is a perfect, and apt description. I can humbly say, without pause, that I do not have nearly the credentials or history with DMT as Dr. Strassman, but I would like to add to the many descriptive terms that could be used to help express the profoundness of this molecule. There are countless colorful adjectives that can easily be used in future books that would also be appropriate; however, throughout my many DMT sessions, I kept saying to myself that "this is a Miracle Molecule." I can say with confidence that this wonderful drug is *both* the Spirit Molecule, and the Miracle Molecule...*and* the list-goes-on molecule.

During my initial DMT session, albeit a pretty intense one, my entire physiological being was instantly reset. Every sensory input that I was exposed to, and every contemplative thought my consciousness generated, was now received, processed, and compartmentalized in a much more effective and efficient way. Self-imposed mental obstacles dissipated, and rehabilitation of the self-inflicted psychic trauma was able to start. DMT answered all the questions, it removed all the fog, and it allowed me to feel complete contentment for the first time in my adult life. It connected me to other dimensional beings and locations, and it allowed me to fully and easily absorb back into the Universal and Absolute field of energy that was the familiar home that I had been unsuccessfully, and desperately, searching for my entire life. And yes...it allowed me to talk to "God," as well as walk with Angels, learn from Aliens, fight with Demons, and manifest physical realities beyond my wildest imaginations. If that is not a Miracle Molecule, then I don't know what is.

DMT, which is short for dimethyltryptamine, is a simple chemical compound that is naturally produced in many plants and animals, including humans. This specific quality, unique among known psychedelics, is one of the leading reasons Dr. Strassman put so much time and effort into a five-year controlled study. He was not only intrigued by the fact that DMT is endogenous, meaning produced within our own bodies, but also by which stages in the human life cycle the body produces large pulses of DMT. There are crucial times shortly after conception, during near-death experiences, and again right before death where the body naturally increases DMT production.

Dr. Strassman not only wanted to understand this correlation better from a medical and scientific standpoint; but due to his appreciation for Eastern religions, meditation, and spirituality, he designed the study with an open mind. He did not dismiss the vivid stories his volunteers shared with him about aliens and God as mere illusions of a hallucinogenic mind, and in fact he purposely provided them with an environment to feel comfortable holding nothing back. He was seeking, or more appropriately, he was allowing for something more profound, and he certainly found it. The data and personal stories that he, his colleagues, and lucky volunteers were able to produce, put DMT back on the map. He forced the medical and spiritual communities to open their eyes to the amazing potential of this now clinically proven "Spirit Molecule." They could no longer turn a blind eye and simply ignore the significance of what he elucidated.

I share Dr. Strassman's opinion that DMT's endogenous quality is what sets it apart from other psychedelics, and why it warrants further investigation. I am quite confident that it is also a significant reason so many people have such an innate affinity to DMT, and why it is so effective at regulating and altering human physiology and perception. It interacts with the body in a similar way to other psychedelics, like psilocybin mushrooms, and even some prescription medications, but the fact that you are not introducing a foreign substance into your body makes it very natural and normal to feel at ease while under its influence. There is a very unique and odd familiarity that you experience with the smell, taste, and feelings that DMT produces. These sensations will be discussed in later chapters, but I wanted to emphasize the fact that DMT is not only a naturally produced molecule, but it is naturally produced *in your own body*.

There is a good amount of literature outlining the chemical structure of DMT, how it is biologically made, where in the body it is produced, and how it is metabolized. There are learned, experienced authors and researchers that have written extensively on the physical and chemical attributes of dimethyltryptamine (Dr. Steven Barker, Dr. Rick Strassman, Dr. Dennis McKenna to name a few). That level of in-depth information is not necessary for what I am trying to convey in this book; however, it is very interesting to the type of mind that is inclined toward that level of detail. I encourage anyone who is curious in personally using DMT to conduct a more thorough investigation of the Miracle Molecule, starting with the names mentioned above.

The limitless potential of the human consciousness, and the life-affirming power of having a properly functioning brain and heart, has been meticulously and beautifully cataloged and expressed through the works of Dr. Joe Dispenza. In his captivating book *Becoming Supernatural*, Dr. Dispenza outlines the processes the body goes through to produce and metabolize molecules in the brain, the importance of the pineal gland, and how controlling the vibrational energy of your mind and body can produce results that are unbelievable, and way beyond mathematical probability. I highly recommend reading this book to help better understand and appreciate the intense physiological responses you will experience when you increase the amounts of DMT your body has access to. Among the many miraculous attributes of DMT that he confirms with his brain scan data is that through meditation and breathing exercises, you can increase the natural levels of DMT within your body to concentrations that are noticeable, and elevated enough to effect a significant change in mood and behavior.

Whether you smoke it, drink it, or manufacture it within your own body, DMT will alter the way you perceive and interact with the world around you. Your brain opens up blocked pathways to allow for the transmission of new information. Your intertwined synapses fire with an increased intensity and connectivity. Your senses become enhanced and hyper-receptive to allow for the expansion of your self-awareness. You will understand with clarity the true source of the power and energy that generates and replenishes your mind, body, and soul.

Experiencing the life-changing effects of a DMT session on your mental, physical, and spiritual well-being will forever change how you navigate your day-to-day life. All of the lingering, unanswered questions that have plagued you in the past get convincingly answered by a higher consciousness. While deep into a DMT session you can have one-on-one conversations with God, Source, Infinite Intelligence, aliens, etc., and no topic is off-limits; all parties are on truth serum, and there are no ulterior motives on either side. You will be able to tap into different dimensions of space and time to find the location, origin, and higher meaning of your most personal and deep inquiries. I am not being dramatic when I say DMT is a life-changer. DMT will inspire miracles to manifest within you, and around you.

CHAPTER 3

Let's Take a Trip:
What a DMT Session Feels Like
and How to Prepare for It

To reap the full benefits of DMT, I would suggest trying both methods of consumption: drinking/eating the liquid brew and smoking/vaping it in crystal form. Both ways of getting the DMT into your system will produce very unique experiences, and both have characteristics that can be useful and/or desired depending on what your intention for the DMT session may be. Whichever path you decide to take, there are two main factors that are essential, and absolutely must be given attention to, in order to have a successful and enjoyable DMT session: 1) take the time to create the perfect environment, and 2) have positive and specific intentions for each session.

Proper preparation will also help avoid a "bad trip," where you become anxious, fearful, or feel unsafe.

The first suggestion may sound pretty basic, but you do not want to learn this lesson the hard way. Priority number one is to properly take care of the physical space and environment in which you will be consuming the Miracle Molecule. This includes the other people or animals that may be in the room, or may walk into that physical space or environment. What you consider a comfortable and safe space is a personal choice, but there are some fundamental conditions you should address to ensure that you feel relaxed and secure:

1. Temperature. Nothing too cold or too hot, because you will become really fucking cold or really fucking hot. You want your body as relaxed and comfortable as possible, and the last thing you want to be is freezing with goosebumps, or sweating your ass off as you are trying to ascend through the phases of this incredible experience.

2. Floor, seat, or bed? Find a comfortable place to be planted and safe, where you can melt your physical body away and feel anchored. You will not have complete control of your body when DMT fully hits you, and you will want to simply "let go," and sink into something soft and supportive.

3. Light or dark? Do you want to experience the hallucinogenic visions with your eyes open, and with light
and color stimulation, or do you want to be in complete darkness and see what wondrous and beautiful
sights and scenes your own consciousness creates?
Both can be fun, enlightening, and intense, but this
should be decided before you start your session.

4. Sounds or silence? Similar to your decision of light
or dark, this one can be extremely stimulating either
way. Calming, soft, and flowing music can add a layer
of complexity to the experience, and if there is a
certain meditative track or song that puts you into a
receptive and positive state of mind, it can help set
the mood in a personal way. It's really just about
being as comfortable as possible, and in a place that
will be supportive of a positive experience.

5. Textures. Whatever you like to touch, have it around.
It can be a plush blanket, a smooth rubbing stone, a
piece of ribbon, soft blades of grass, etc. Your mind
will be off doing its own thing, and it helps ground
you to have something familiar to feel in your hands,
especially as you are coming down.

Once the physical space and environment is set up to
your liking, it is now time to address the other important
matter that you must take care of. It is crucial that you are

mindful, and set your intention and goals for each DMT journey you are about take. This is not some hippy-dippy, esoteric, high-level quantum theory, law of attraction bullshit. Actually, yes, it is! Believe that "bullshit" or not, you *Do Not* want to drink DMT brew or smoke DMT crystals if you are in a negative, pissed off, aggressive, or low vibrational state of mind. This is how you prevent the proverbial "bad trip." I recommend being in such states as gratitude, contentment, open-mindedness, love, acceptance, joy, etc.

It is like walking into a movie theater and choosing between a gory indie horror movie, or an animated Disney comedy. There may be times when you want to see the death and destruction flick, but may I suggest that you start off your initial DMT experiences with the warm and fuzzy movies that end with "happily ever after." After a few experiences, and perhaps if you are feeling adventurous, you can move on to one of the smaller theaters where there is just that one creepy guy sitting in the back row enjoying the carnage on the screen. (I have been *that* creepy guy in the back row, and believe me, the movies they play in those smaller theaters at the end of the hallway will mess with your head. Do not buy a ticket to this type of show unless you are prepared for what you are about to watch.) In summary, be in a good mental state and physical place where you can be relaxed and fully experience the life-changing molecule that you are about to enjoy.

There are several differences in how your body responds to a DMT brew session versus a DMT crystal session. The most significant is the time needed to break down the molecule. Any psychedelic experience is going to be very intimate and subjective, and inherently will be difficult to accurately and succinctly describe. I will do my best to at least set some expectations or guidelines to help anticipate what you may encounter on this transformative journey. After just a few DMT sessions you will become very comfortable with the sensations you feel, and the different dimensions you will explore. You will figure out what works for you, what does not, and simply what "feels good." Follow what your own body tells you, and don't be afraid to play around with different environmental settings, dosages, methods, etc. What is appropriate for me may not be appropriate for someone else, and I can honestly say that every time I have used DMT, I have learned something new.

The honest answer to what the proper dose of DMT brew is: it is different for everyone, and it depends on a lot of factors. Think along the lines of how different people's tolerances can be with alcohol, and perhaps even more appropriate, the difference in tolerance levels to homemade moonshine where the proof percentage is only approximately known. There will be quite the variation in tolerance levels between someone that weighs 150 lbs. and someone that weighs 250 lbs., between someone that rarely (or never) drinks and someone that has several beverages a day, between someone who has recently eaten a large meal and someone who has not eaten all day, between someone who is taking certain types of prescription medication that create adverse side effects and someone who is not. Each different batch of brew that you make will also have its own unique characteristics and strengths that will have to be "figured out" by experimenting, and seeing how your body responds.

One of the more important factors in determining the proper dosage, is your personal intention or goal for that particular session. Are you micro dosing to make your Sunday housecleaning more enjoyable, or are you hoping to blast between astral planes, converse with gods, relive past life reincarnations, and find the answers to questions like "Who the Fuck Am I?"? The necessary quantities of DMT will clearly be much different depending on what you are trying to accomplish.

This is my personal experience consuming DMT brew. For context I am a forty-two-year-old male, five feet ten inches, 180 lbs. in relatively good health, active, who does not take any prescription drugs or drink alcohol. I followed the general recipe guidelines that are provided later in this book, and every time produced a brew that was extremely strong. When micro dosing, I would typically either just take a small "shot" straight up, or add a couple of ounces to a cup of coffee or smoothie. This will allow for a slow onset of relatively mild changes in perception and sensory interpretation. It will take the edge off, but still allow you to engage and interact with people, complete tasks, create art, enjoy physical actively, etc., and will not last more than an hour or so.

The whole concept of "micro" dosing is that you are *not* taking a full dose, or even half a dose for that matter. The goal is to take just enough DMT so that your body and mind feel the effects without losing control of either. If you desire to be in this slightly altered state for a prolonged period of time, consuming several micro doses throughout the day can keep you at a nice, even, and controllable level of elated bliss. If you are new to DMT, I would I highly recommend starting off with an overabundance of caution. You should not drink a twelve-pack of beer if you have never had a beer before—it probably will not leave you with a positive memory of the experience—and you should similarly not drink a massive jug of DMT brew if it is your first time.

A "full" dose of DMT brew is a whole different story! A full dose requires a bit more planning, and the previous suggestions about being conscious of your physical space, environment, and intention are critical. When looking to have a more profound experience, I would typically drink one to two cups within a thirty-minute period. The effects become noticeable pretty quickly, and you will not be sitting there waiting for something to happen. It will be very obvious that you just ingested a psychedelic molecule, and now it is time to sit back and enjoy the show. Your body needs some time to fully metabolize and absorb the liquid or solid that has been consumed, so even though you start feeling the sensations pretty quickly, this process will take several hours to play out. Full intensity will typically take about an hour, and there is a pretty consistent crescendo to the peak, which can last a couple hours or more. Coming down is pretty uneventful and kind of just happens. I have never experienced any physical illness or discomfort when coming back to "normal," but there is a sense of sadness and melancholy that you are leaving behind your "true" self, and that the "normal" world you are coming back to is not really "reality."

This would be the proper time to bring up...throwing up, which can happen shortly after ingesting DMT brew. Do you sometimes throw up when you drink/eat DMT brew? Yes. Do you throw up every time? No. If you throw up, does that mean you will have, or are having a "bad trip"? No. If you do not throw up, does that mean you did not take enough, and should take more? No. That being said, the ideal scenario is that you experiment and discover what volumes and/or rates of consumption work best for you. Ideally you find what allows for the most intense session, without making yourself go through the never pleasant process of retching your guts out multiple times.

With a DMT brew session (as opposed to when you smoke the crystals), you get to kind of ease your way into a very intense situation. As your body slides into the full experience, your vision will start to become more focused, while at the same time start to pick up peripheral movement of objects that are beginning to distort and blend together. There is not so much of the chaotic kaleidoscopic display that you have with smoking the crystals, but the air around you is transmuted into a viscous liquid that you can move and manipulate with your hands. It becomes natural to swirl, play with, and control the stream-like currents of energy that you can now texturally feel all around you. The visuals when ingesting DMT stay more consistent and calmer than in the jaw-dropping pandemonium of sights and sounds that occur when you smoke DMT.

There is a low and pleasant hum or ringing that provides a consistent background noise to let you know that your brain is vibrating at higher frequencies. Time becomes a laughable illusion, and you comfortably realize that you are just drifting in some sort of universal current where there is just the simple and absolute "now." The bullshit in the past and the bullshit in the future do not exist. There is only what is in front of you that matters, or more accurately, there is only what you are "in the middle of" that matters.

If you spend the time setting up your environment properly, this is when you begin to deeply contemplate everything you look at, hear, feel, and perceive. What would normally be subconscious thoughts that you dismiss by habit, become loud statements and questions that are blasted forcefully into the omniscient matrix of the Universe. Your cerebral vibrations are received and answered by forces and beings that were previously not accessible through concentration alone. Once you are in this euphoric state, my experience is one of three things will happen:

1. You will simply sit back and enjoy the show. You are comfortable, relaxed, and content. You are interested in exploring the environment you have set up, and have fun trying to process the new sensory information you are receiving. You are in awe of the beauty radiating around you and from within you. You are watching the program, not really directing it. You are chilling....and are happy doing it.

2. You realize very quickly that you have a unique opportunity to get the answers to any question you ask. Your subconscious thoughts are being loudly projected, *unfiltered*, into the vastness of your now hyper-astute consciousness. These thoughts race out into the unknown ether to find their source, solution, and proper perspective. What answers back, and gives you the most profound information, is simply and profoundly *You. You* instantly answer all of *your* own questions with brutal honesty, lightning speed, and unwavering clarity. You provide yourself with the revelations and epiphanies you are seeking, and

are satisfied as to the credentials and authority of the person in the mirror who provided the insight.

3. Repeat everything I said in option number 2, however, what answers back is distinctly *Not You!* This is where shit can get kind of funky. (I can only imagine how Dr. Strassman must have felt to process the information he gathered from listening to all of the stories of his volunteers, then presenting this information his professional colleagues!). I have conversed with Gods, with Demons, with Angels, with Spirits, with Sights, with Sounds, and with frequencies of energies that I simply do not have the scientific background or vocabulary to accurately describe. When getting towards the end of your session and your non-DMT senses are returning, you pretty much just shake your head in awe and try to internalize what just took place.

The effects of smoking DMT crystals are similar, but more intense, and short-lived compared to that produced by a DMT brew session, only lasting about ten minutes or so. You can smoke DMT out of a marijuana pipe, a specialized "crystal" pipe, use a vape pen with a setup for shatter and/or resin, or make your own vape cartridge. Any method will work just fine, but I did find that using the vape pen was more conservative, efficient, and easy. The vape pen is suggested if you want to take multiple, deep hits, and are looking to have a prolonged and somewhat regulated transformative experience. The vape pen also provides and allows for easy storage and/or transport, and will prevent you from having a precious glob of DMT wastefully burning in your pipe while you hold in the hit you just took.

If you do use a normal style pipe, make sure you put some marijuana, tobacco, or other herb in the pipe first to act as a screen, and have something to cap it off to prevent the smoke from escaping between hits. Do not use your finger; the burning glob of DMT will stick to it. Learn from my mistake. Most vape stores and/or head shops will have the specialized "crystal" pipes or bongs, and I recommend getting one of these setups if you plan on adding DMT to your self-preservation and maintenance schedule. These style pipes are great for taking large hits and pushing your experience and tolerance to the limits.

How much DMT you "need" to smoke, once again, depends on what your intention for the session is. Micro dosing DMT crystal is kind of an oxymoron, but it can be done. Even one hit will drastically alter your state of being, but if you if take relatively small hits, or use the vape pen on a lower setting, you can kind of throttle your DMT intake to provide pleasant mental and physical sensations without having the mind-blowing, "holy shit" experience. How much DMT crystal you need weight wise, or how many hits it will require to have a full-blown DMT experience is something you must figure out for yourself. Normally about four or five deep hits will provide for a very profound experience; taking a few more hits will allow for something magical. If smoking the crystals in a pipe, I typically add the equivalent volume of about two or three peppercorns or BBs for a standard session, and the equivalent of about four or five peppercorns or BBs for a deeper session. Whether using a pipe or a vape pen, I find that when I reach a DMT saturation point that allows for the deepest, most mystical, and most transcendental sessions, there is a distinct nasal cavity sensation, combined with a soft palate reflex that tells me it is time to sit back and enjoy the next ten minutes.

My personal story smoking DMT crystals is probably not going be like most others, and I would not necessarily suggest you follow my path exactly. I want to share my experience because I think it is important for the scientific community, as well as potential DMT users, to have as much information on dosing as possible. Please remember, I was in a very unique mental place, and I was also very comfortable and familiar with other psychedelics like shrooms and acid. I was approaching this session as if it were a scientific experiment. I was confident my mind could handle whatever was to come, and honestly, at that point in my life, I could not give two shits if my brain exploded.

My first DMT crystal session took place in the perfect physical space and environment. I was welcomed into a close friend's home, and I was 100 percent comfortable, at ease, and protected. My intention, although of a positive nature, was pretty extreme and excessive, and I was not leaving until I had the answers to my internal conflicts. I was also fortunate that I was not limited in the amount of crystals I was able to smoke, and I had the perfect vape pen set up.

Within about an hour and a half, I took about fifty massive hits of DMT. Before you call "bullshit," let me break down how it went. First session, I took two hits and immediately felt it, took two more and sat back and tried to internalize what was happening. What initially struck me as odd, was how familiar the taste and smell of DMT was. I innately, and quickly, felt that I was not in any danger, even though the physical world in front of my eyes was performing a cosmic dance to a song I had never heard before. I was in awe and thoroughly impressed by my initial introduction to DMT, but I did not have any enlightening revelations.

My friend and I had prepared for a scientific experiment, and I *was* the disposable lab rat, so now that I was comfortable with the feeling of DMT pulsing through my body, we could let the real data collection begin. (Cue the sinister and ominous laughter.) Now, I do not want to causally gloss over the glorious sensory inputs and vibrations that I felt during those first few minutes, but I want to make sure you understand how the math of the number of hits works out, so please bear with me, and I will get to back to the *Alice in Wonderland* scenery shortly.

The next five sessions all took place roughly ten minutes apart from one another. Second session, I pushed it a
bit further and took six or seven massive hits. Third session, another six or seven massive hits. Fourth session, six
or seven massive hits. Fifth session, six or seven massive
hits. Sixth session, six or seven massive hits. By this time,
roughly an hour has gone by, and my friend (now shaman)
is getting a bit concerned that I am trying to overdo it or
hurt myself, but he intimately knows my story and mental
struggles, and allows me to continue my journey, while
continuing to provide me with nothing but positive
energy and love.

As absolutely insane as the last hour of my life just
was, I still did not have my answers, nor did I see or
talk to any entities or spirits or aliens. I was feeling like
a punch-drunk boxer running on instinct (remember,
DMT is endogenous, so it could very well be *instinc-
tual*), but I knew the Universe was about to give up and
go down for the count. Infinite Intelligence would even-
tually puke up the answers I was seeking, I just had to
prove I was a worthy opponent who was willing and
able to go the distance, and not quit in the last round. I
positively reinforced my intentions, and approached the
next (and last) session with a sense of genuine appreciation for what was already exposed and unveiled to me. I
made a simple and sincere "ask" of the Universe, and then
I jumped off the cliff.

My seventh session I took eight or nine massive hits,

and I instantly knew *that* was the last session for the day. It started off like the others, but then took a very different turn. The crazy visual hallucinations dulled, the humming buzz quieted, and my entire being became magnetically charged and pulled in all directions at the same time. I floated in a state of Nirvana. My eyes rolled upward in my head and started twitching. That's when "something" communicated with me. This conveyance of information was *not* my mind or body playing tricks on me, nor me simply being messed up on drugs. I had just spent the last hour engaged in that game, and was very familiar with what that felt like. This was neither my own consciousness, nor subconscious ramblings. I was acutely aware of the power, impact, and sound of those as well; they had been driving me crazy for the last two years of my life.

The communication I received during this session was unique, and affected me unlike anything I had ever experience before. This communication came from Source, God, Infinite Intelligence, etc., and it instantly reset my entire being. Even though I had just consumed a very large of dose of DMT, as soon as I got "my answer," I came back to my non-DMT senses (I refuse to call them my "normal" senses) and crumbled into a crying mess on my friend's living room floor. My tears were not ones of sadness, nor of joy for that matter, but big ol' tears of gratitude. I had been cruelly trapped in my own mental maze for most of my adult life, and now I knew in every atom of my being that my struggle was *all* an illusion. I was not only handed the set of keys to unlock the doors that I had previously been trying to kick down, but I was given the master key to unlock any door I may ever want to open in the future. That was the first of many times that I said to myself "That's a Miracle Molecule!"

Since that miraculous day, I have used DMT hundreds of times as an integral part of my meditation and spiritual growth practices, as well as to aid in my ability to induce lucid dreaming, have a tantric connection with my body and those of my sexual partners, and stay mindful and present in my daily activities.

Each session, the sensations you experience and lessons you learn will be unique, and will build upon knowledge gained in the previous session. You will most likely not have an epiphany *every* time you use DMT, but I guarantee that you *will* have them, and all you need is one to save your life and put you on the right path. A majority of the time, you will have experiences more like mine in sessions two through six: a ten-minute blast followed by an hour of intense contemplation. That blast, and what it looks, sounds, and feels like is up to you. You have to take the time to physically and mentally prepare for this journey.

You are the composer, the conductor, and the orches-tra. You are the architect, the builder, and the interior designer. You are the farmer, the chef, and the waitress. Use whatever analogy resonates with you, but if you want to see an entertaining show, in a beautiful old building and enjoy an incredible meal it takes some effort and planning. DMT will take you to the dinner show of your choice, so make sure you choose the venue and the ticket you purchase wisely. Don't complain if you are seated next to the kitchen, behind a structural column with no view, sitting next to a douche bag, at a show you hate, about to be served a shitty meal. You can float in Heaven, or you can fester in Hell. Red pill or blue pill?

An individual can experience the euphoric effects of dimethyltryptamine through meditation, and/or breathing exercises, and it is a powerful and personal accomplishment that is worth pursuing. Admittedly, not as sensorily stimulating as that of a full dose of brew or crystals, but perhaps even more gratifying. The importance of your intention is beautifully on display when you feel DMT in this manner. Taking the personal time out of your busy day to relax, shut out all of the distractions, and simply breathe and meditate is essential to being mentally healthy. By calming your internal thoughts, and consciously focusing on the energy you are breathing into and out of your body, you can stimulate your pineal gland to "get you high."

The feelings and emotions you experience during this type of DMT session are uniquely special. Gratitude and contentment swirl with bliss and joy, as your vibrational frequency blends effortlessly with that of the Universe, all while deep in a meditative state. It is Heaven, it is

Nirvana, it is the velvety soft feel of grace, and it is created intentionally within your own consciousness. Do a
few of these types of DMT sessions, and you will understand why "Miracle Molecule" kept emanating from my
thoughts. You can learn to do this in an afternoon, just ask
DMT and the Universe for guidance (and watch a few
videos of proven methods from qualified teachers to seal
the deal).

CHAPTER 4

Transcendental Sex, Art, and Science: DMT in the Bedroom, Art Studio, and Research Lab

ONE OF THE MOST GLORIOUS ATTRIBUTES OF DIMETH-yltryptamine is that it is a fast-acting catalyst that can be utilized to set off beautiful cascades of novel, profound, and fascinating mental and physical experiences. Whether it is endogenously produced by meditation, or smoked/ingested, the bedroom, art studio, and research lab are locations where the benefits of this molecule need to be explored to their utmost limits.

As mentioned in previous chapters, setting your intention and providing the proper environment are crucial components to fully exploiting all of the miraculous qualities of DMT. The potential for rapturous pleasure and innovative insight generated by having your sensory inputs and outputs wildly increased and enhanced will make enjoying sex, creating art, and conducting scientific studies all the more enjoyable and productive. These areas of human endeavor are where properly understanding the beneficial effects of DMT can help expand what is currently known; not only within an individual's consciousness, but also within collective human consciousness as a whole.

The ability to observe your mind, body, and soul with fresh synaptic pathways, new physiological awareness, and instant connectivity to the Universal field of energy and information, will allow for a wonderous expansion of thought, and subsequent expression of ideas. The short duration of the psychedelic portion of a DMT trip allows for multiple sessions over a period of just a few hours, and allows for a unique opportunity to process, calibrate, and compartmentalize the instruction and intelligence gained from the new dimensions of conscious awareness that is accessible while under the influence of this amazing drug. The tantric sex master, creative genius, and curious researcher all have something to learn, experience, and gain by exploring the boundless potential and timeless wisdom that is contained within these higher levels of vibrational thought.

Sex on DMT is mind-blowing, and brings the euphoria and ecstasy of intense sexual interactions to a whole new level. For the sake of science, and as a requirement to write this chapter, I had to have a lot of sex, and smoke a lot of DMT. When I decided to become an author, I knew I would have to make some sacrifices, and these were two I was willing to make. If there is any occasion to really make sure to take care of intention and environment, this would be the time. It is extremely important to have a thorough and open-minded conversation as to what each partner may or may not experience, and to what actions they may or may not want to partake in. I am extremely fortunate to have an ideal sexual partner, unlimited DMT, and the perfect environment to conduct my research. (I am very happy I did not off myself out in the desert.)

My first experience did not go as planned, but still ended beautifully. I will avoid graphic details; however, I do want to share what I have learned to help anyone seeking this information. The "plan" was that during intercourse, I would take several hits and try to climax during the intense couple of minutes that DMT first starts taking effect. What actually happened is that as soon as I took my multiple hits, all the blood and mental focus rushed from below my waist up to my brain, and I lost my erection. My attention went down a myriad of uncontrollable tangential paths in an attempt to process all of sights, sounds, smells, feelings, and emotions that were all instantaneously amplified and exploding throughout my body. My partner understood exactly what to do, and seamlessly made the next few minutes about being grounded, secure, and loved. I was able to see the pure and natural beauty radiating from her soul, and I knew I was exactly where I needed and wanted to be. We continued talking and touching each other as I went through the phases of my trip. After about ten minutes or so I was able to get the blood back to where I needed it to be, and we continued on to have a satisfying evening.

My sexual partner is also one of my DMT research partners, so we processed the data we had collected and came up with ideas for the next session. The biggest difference was our intention. Instead of trying to go for insane sensory fireworks, and attempting to synchronize climax of orgasm with climax of DMT trip, we decided to go for a more long and steady approach, and focused on enjoying the journey. Instead of taking five or six big hits, then laying back and melting into the bed and waiting for something to happen, we decided to work smaller, continual doses into a prolonged sexual experience.

We began by concentrating on pleasing the other person. This personally allowed me to not worry about if I was keeping an erection or not, and to just focus on the energy I was sharing with the woman that I was with, and was making love to. This is where DMT unlocked an unexpected bonus. With heightened DMT senses and intuition, I was able to intimately experience her body responding to my touch in an entirely new way. I could feel her heart rapidly pumping blood, hear her lungs absorbing oxygen, and I could consume her essence with an arousing new clarity of what I was capable of doing to her body. We were able to effortlessly synchronize our involuntary muscle spasms, and we were able to connect at a cellular and vibrational level that took us each to previously unknown levels of pleasure and stimulation. The concern of being able to stay hard quickly dissipated, and was replaced with a mutual confidence that our bodies were so locked into what our intentions were, that the night was only going to continue to get more intense and amazing.

Orgasm was inevitable, so we decided to get into "science data collection mode" and simply enjoy each prolonged and engorged second of nirvana and state of bliss that we were both in. We were able to hand off the vape pen back and forth as we engaged and intertwined with one another. We gave each other shotgun hits while kissing, visually penetrating each other's psyches with our newly expanded eyes. It was like we were having a threesome with God, and they were showing us the techniques to fully experience the human body through sexual expression. Needless to say, DMT is now an important part of not only our sexual relationship and routine, but also has increased the trust and love we have for one another. We know that we have experienced something very few couples have ever experienced, and we felt it in the core of every atom of our beings. We had transcendental sex.

DMT can be an important stimulant, and in some cases, a necessary savior in the bedroom for couples in all stages of their relationships. Depending on what is desired, DMT can ignite the spark, sustain the blaze, or ensure the explosion. It is my theory, based on the many personal experiences of myself and partner, that the body pulses a large dose of endogenous DMT right before and during sexual climax. On many occasions we have tasted and smelled DMT at these moments of sexual excitement with no external DMT being used or present. I would love to donate my body to science for this study if there is any academic interest and ability to test my theory out.

Creating art, during and after a DMT session, will undoubtedly provide the world with beautiful and mind-blowing representations from the artist's hallucinogenic visions. I have always loved and admired Alex Grey's amazing talent to produce art that transcends what most humans could ever imagine, let alone put on a canvas or screen. His art immediately comes to mind when writing this chapter. His ability to "see" beyond what normal human senses typically allow is one of the reasons his work resonates with millions of people. If you have not seen any of his work, please take a moment to look him up. His creations are the closest to a visual representation of a DMT trip that I have seen yet.

I am certainly no Alex Grey, but I do express myself artistically through several mediums, and I can tell you firsthand that properly harnessing the power of DMT will help break through any creative block an artist may be going through. It can give them direct access to a dimensional space and energy where they can innately and joyfully tap into the state of "flow" that all artists crave and seek. It is in this meditative mental state that many artists produce their most profound and personally important work. DMT allows for the artist's mind to easily receive insight and inspiration from beyond the normal realms of conscious thought.

If one considers an artist to be a student and translator of how the world works, then the artist who has access to DMT has access to the greatest master and mentor of all time. They can get one-on-one lessons from "The Artist" that created the Universe itself! All they have to do is ask nicely, and take a couple of hits of DMT. The art that is influenced by this omniscient instructor is by definition "transcendental," and I for one want to see more of it.

Enjoying artwork created by others, during and after a DMT session, will also provide for quite the enlightening experience. As mentioned in previous chapters, DMT resets, rewires, and upgrades your entire suite of sensory software. If you think Alex Grey's work is visually stimulating through the lens of your normal sensory perception, just imagine what it will look like wearing DMT-colored glasses. The immediate effect on your visual senses is probably the most noticeable effect that DMT has on your body.

On the day of my first session, I remember saying that

I "saw new colors and new shapes." Not necessarily the most articulate description, but it points to the foundational change in how you will experience your exterior environment and internal visions. To try to paint a more accurate picture of what you may see and experience when enjoying visual art, and to save hundreds of inadequate words trying to describe the indescribable, I ask the reader again to look up the work of Alex Grey and/ or several of his talented contemporaries, whether it be in traditional media forms, or computer-generated digital art.

DMT will overlay this psychedelic style and depth of complexity on anything you focus your attention on. There is a stimulating kaleidoscopic movement and morphing of iridescent colors, shapes, and patterns that is both fluid and chaotic at the same time. The shifts in visual perception occur in dramatic pulses, connected by continually morphing transitions that appear to be manipulated by powers beyond our present understanding. I have come to term this motion the "cosmic twitch" and it appears to be random, yet also possess a universal intelligence and coherence.

The distinction between central and peripheral vision fades, and you develop a 360-degree point of view that is both infinite and microscopic at the same time. Spatial perspective is uniquely NOT three-dimensional, and there is no separation between the "seen" and the "seer." The optical illusions of your "normal" state get quickly replaced with the optical realities of your more authentic and expanded DMT state. Like the surreal visions one remembers from a lucid dream, the images one sees while saturated with DMT will have a lasting impression that will influence how you interpret the information your brain supplies you with for the rest of your life. What you have seen in the depths of a DMT trip cannot be unseen, and that is just the way you will prefer it.

Listening to music is also contemplated and enjoyed in a vastly enhanced way. Whether the music is created by a human being, another living creature, Mother Nature, or the internal hum and cadence generated by your own consciousness, you will process and absorb sound vibrations in a more comprehensive way once the muffling filters have been removed by DMT. Your favorite songs are received with a startling new clarity, and you will gain the ability to truly appreciate the complexity of the composition as the artist intended. What you previously heard as four instruments playing a bass line and hook is now ten instruments and a synthesizer seamlessly tying half a dozen harmonic flows together. Those catchy lyrics that you never really understood become philosophic prose that resonates with you to your core. You gain the ability fade in or out, and/or focus on specific aspects of the song that you never even noticed before.

DMT amplifies natural melodies such as the mating songs of birds and bugs, and allows you to appreciate and feel the seduction. The soothing sound waves produced by Mother Nature, in the pulse of her water and the breath of her wind, synergistically combine with the beat of your heart, and the pace of your breathing. You obtain the ability to effortlessly quiet the bullshit internal noise of your mind that previously had prevented you from hearing the Universal symphony as its Composer intended. Similar to seeing new shapes and colors, new frequencies and patterns are now acknowledged by your auditory structures.

One of the most profound abilities I was able to procure through the use of DMT was the ability to appreciate the sound of silence. Sitting in a soundless room, you are able perceive the ticks, clicks, and beats of the cosmos, but the real fun comes when you cup your ears with your hands and listen to the "silence" of your mind. Terence McKenna, one of the original gangster psychonauts and psychedelic teachers who was a huge proponent of DMT, used the phrase "the voice of our own DNA" in an interview as a beautiful way to describe this frequency. The first time I truly listened to the creation and contemplation of my own thoughts, I was blown away. I was unaware that I could conduct such a beautiful concert. I felt like I was a DJ, and had God's playlist full of songs and sounds to scratch and mix as desired.

Art and individual creativity in general are expressed through countless different means and mediums, and DMT has the potential to permeate every aspect of how we experience all of them. In the kitchen, the chef's palate and sense of smell can become even more worldly and acute, allowing for even more mouthwatering masterpieces to be created. On the sports field, in the ocean, or on the mountain, athletes will be able to hone their skills more naturally and quickly due to the increased coherence between mind and body. Without fear, the engineer will push the limits of what is allowed by physics in our 3D world because she understands the laws that govern higher dimensions. The fly fisherman will hand spin the most eloquent of lures, the creative writer will craft their magnum opus, the sculptor will carve his exact vision, all with a little extra flair and confidence due to the transcendent source of their inspiration: the Miracle Molecule DMT. For the person who is doing the creating, DMT throws rocket fuel on your creative spark. For the person who is doing the enjoying, DMT brings you to the show by limousine, gives you front row seats and backstage passes, and sends you home with an autographed poster from the entire cast of the production.

Transcendent sex should be on everybody's bucket list, and transcendent art should be the ambition of every artist; however, transcendent science has the potential to heal our wounded planet and save lives. Transcendent science is the realm where the Miracle Molecule can really shine. There are several fields of study like quantum physics, epigenetics, artificial intelligence, mental health, neuroplasticity and neurogenesis, autism, etc., where a fresh perspective could be all that is needed to have that breakthrough "ah-ha!" moment. It only takes a handful of great scientific minds to significantly alter and accelerate each one of these areas of research.

In addition to the sensory upgrades that DMT provides, the increased clarity of intuition and ability to interpret new information are where the real excitement lies. Scientific method and repetitious procedure are certainly important, but they have their limitations when pushing the boundaries of empirical thought. I am not necessarily suggesting that scientists and researchers pass a vape pen back and forth in the middle of conducting their investigations and analysis, but I am extremely confident that there are huge benefits to be gained by this specific caste of thinkers by partaking in sessions of DMT, followed by sessions of quiet contemplation and reflection. The DMT-boosted ability of these men and women to connect and understand the proverbial dots, as well as see beyond the walls of conventional logic, will exponentially increase their unique aptitudes and scientific faculties. Their bolstered awareness of the Universal thread that binds together every sentient being to each other and its Source will infuse and enrich the research with empathy and sympathy that is much needed if we are to stop the self-destructive path that the human species is currently on. Scientific minds that have been influenced by DMT may be what are needed to prepare our species for the transformative (and transcendental) next step in our evolution.

In a perfect world, the following paragraph would discuss the implications dimethyltryptamine could have on politics. If there is any group of people that could benefit from an altruistic-mindset-inducing Ayahuasca or DMT session, it is politicians. Unfortunately, many of today's policymakers and world leaders appear to be extremely self-centered, egotistical, narcissistic, and petty. DMT would dissolve these limiting and small-minded personality traits, and smack the smug smirk right off their faces. The desire (and ability) to cooperate with one another, tolerate differing opinions, and blend practical ideas for the common good of "the people" would be a natural side effect of the inspiring interconnectedness they experienced while deep in the realms of DMT saturation. DMT could expose these individuals to a dose of Universal understanding that would be a great foundation to build policies off of. I will share my stash if any politicians are ready for a session.

CHAPTER 5

Grandma's Recipe:
How to Make Your Own DMT

Another one of the miraculous qualities of
dimethyltryptamine is that anyone can easily make it; however, that does not mean that everyone *should*. Before we
get into grandma's recipe, let me please channel my inner
grandma to make a necessary suggestion: reread the disclaimer at the beginning of this book. Do not do anything
illegal, dangerous, or stupid! You could end up in jail, dead,
or hurting someone. This is not a "recreational drug" that
you should be selling, or nonchalantly sharing with people.
DMT is rocket fuel for the psyche, and it can just as easily
blow up the vessel as it can propel it into outer space.

That being said, humans have been extracting and
using DMT (or producing it endogenously through meditation) for thousands of years. There are dozens of recipes

that can be found in ancient manuscripts, academic publications, and simple online searches. DMT recipe information is readily available to anyone that is looking for it, the materials needed to produce it are inexpensive to buy, and the extraction process is relatively easy and safe. A basic understanding of chemistry and the ability to follow instructions are all that is needed. There are certain ingredients that can be harmful if misused, like sodium hydroxide (NaOH, sold as household drain cleaner called lye) and naphtha (sold as paint or stain thinner), but with proper precautions taken, the following recipes are very easy to replicate.

Determining which material(s) you need to make your personal batch depends on if you want to make a liquid to drink/ingest, or if you want to make crystals to smoke/vape. The source of DMT that you purchase can originate from a variety of plant species, and is sold as raw bark, dried leaves, and/or as concentrates. The laws surrounding the legality of having these products shipped to you depend on where you live. Do your due diligence. Online searches will expose you to several companies that will mail these products discreetly to any address you choose. Pick the one that you feel the most comfortable doing business with, and don't buy more than you need for personal use. Common plants used for extraction that have some of the highest known concentrations of DMT and are available commercially are *Mimosa hostilis*, *Acacia confusa*, and *Psychotria viridis*. Any one of, or a combination of, these plants will give you the base organic material needed to make your own DMT. The secondary ingredients needed to complete the recipe depend on what form of DMT you want to produce; however, all of the products are easily obtainable.

The simplest recipes are ones that make a liquid that you can either drink or use for cooking. You are basically making a version of Ayahuasca, which is a South American hallucinogenic drink used and administered by shamans for spiritual and ceremonial purposes. I liken the process to brewing homemade beer. There are multiple styles of beers, with multiple strengths, and they are made using a bunch of different additives for an assortment of reasons. What is good or bad beer, or weak or strong beer, or how much is a normal serving is a personal opinion, but the basic ingredients of all beer are the same: water, yeast, hops, and malt. Once you have the main recipe down, and know the role each ingredient plays, you can then confidently brew a simple, basic beer. From this foundational beer, you can create endless combinations of strengths and flavor profiles. The malt produces the sugar needed for the yeast to break down into alcohol. The water provides the base liquid, and the hops and other additives provide the complex flavor, color, and viscosity profiles. Making a DMT brew should be approached with the same understanding of the fundamentals, as well as an open mind and the freedom to add your own personal touches.

The main difference between making a DMT brew and a homemade beer is that fermentation is needed to produce the desired amount of alcohol in beer, whereas with a DMT brew, it is a simple extraction process and a matter of concentrations and ratios. Other than choosing which plant species to use as the source of DMT, the other key ingredient(s) you must select is which source of MAOI is added. MAOI stands for monoamine oxidase inhibitor, and there are several readily available products that can be added to your brew to give the needed amounts.

Just as it is crucial to understand what roles malt and yeast play in producing alcohol, and subsequently how buzzed or drunk you get, it is equally important to understand the role that MAOIs play in experiencing a DMT session. The main concept to grasp is this: there is an enzyme in the human brain called monoamine oxidase, and this enzyme is responsible for removing neurotransmitters like serotonin and dopamine, which are chemically and structurally very similar to DMT, from brain tissue. In our particular topic of discussion, the presence and concentration of the MAOI is a major factor in the intensity and length of the DMT session.

The MAOI "inhibits," as the name implies, monoamine oxidase from doing its job. If monoamine oxidase is inhibited, then more of the DMT is able to be experienced for a prolonged period of time. When you ingest DMT, it will be quickly broken down unless a MAOI is

added to slow the process. Very simply, the addition of
the MAOI allows for a longer, more intense experience;
and without it, your brew will be incomplete, and will
not produce the desired psychedelic effects. Common
MAOIs used to make brew are *Banisteriopsis caapi* (which
is what is used in traditional Ayahuasca and can typically
be purchased from the same store that you get the DMT
plant material), Syrian rue, kava kava, black pepper, tur-
meric, and green tea. Concentrated forms of harmine
crystals can also be used. (Please note that literature on
MAOIs indicate that several adverse effects can occur in
combination with certain medications, and proper due
diligence is suggested if you have any concerns).

Making the brew is a pretty straightforward process.
You can use either the bark or leaves, or a combination
of both, of any of the plant species that were mentioned
earlier to supplement the DMT. There are quite a few
options to choose from as far as a base plant material, and
there are studies available that show the relative concentrations. My personal experience with making DMT
brew is using the plants mentioned in this book, which
according to the studies I reviewed are the ones with the
highest concentrations. The information provided in the
product descriptions of each plant species on the various
websites where these materials can be purchased is also
very helpful for picking out your ingredients. Depending
on how you buy your plant base material, you may need
to grind it up using a coffee grinder or food processor

to create the maximum surface area for the extraction process to occur. If bark is being used, you want it to be a consistency similar to loose-leaf tea or large coffee grounds. It can be ground up finer, but obviously it will have to be strained by a finer mesh screen. A pour-over cone-shaped coffee filter works well if the material is very fine. If leaves are being used, you can just break them up and throw them into the brew as is.

Once you have the DMT plant material(s) properly ground up, and have selected which MAOIs to use (each time I made DMT brew, I use a combination of several plant bases and MAOIs), the only other ingredients you will need are quality water (distilled if possible) as your base liquid, and any other herbs, teas, extracts, etc., that you desire to add for flavor or other health benefits. The taste of just the bark/leaves is honestly disgusting! It is worse than shroom tea or a cheap shot of whiskey, and has a distinct bitterness that takes a bit to get used to. I have added things like chai tea, cinnamon, clove, coffee, honey, hibiscus, ashwagandha, peppermint, etc., to help make it a bit more palatable.

The recipes that I came across had quite a bit of variation in the ratios of ingredients, and used approximate measurements for the amounts of each category of additive. Even less was agreed upon when it comes to proper dosing. I think it would now be helpful to switch from using homemade beer as a reference, and now consider the similarities between home-brewed coffee when it comes to ratios and strength. Some people make a pot of coffee with half of a scoop, and some use two scoops. Each amount will produce a pot of coffee, but obviously one will have a much stronger flavor profile, and a higher concentration of caffeine. I use the rough guidelines of 1.5 gallons of water, 2 cups of DMT base plant material, 1 cup of MAOI inhibitor material, then add the flavors and/or other herbs to taste. If concentrates are being used, then adjust amounts as needed. Tweaking these ratios in either direction is certainly allowed and encouraged to fit personal preferences. (Some people like strong espresso black, some like weak coffee with milk and sugar.) The 1.5 gallons of water will reduce to less than a gallon of water, and the actual volume remaining will depend on how long you boil the brew, as well as if you do additional water flushes of the brewing material.

Please note, the boiling process will produce a very distinct, strong, and acrid smell. I recommend boiling either outside or in a well-ventilated area, and away from other people or pets. This is not a recipe you make inside a large apartment complex, dorm building, or in your grandma's kitchen.

Cooking guidelines are as follows:

- Take 0.5 gallons of water and keep aside for flushing of the material after the initial boiling.

- Take 1 gallon of water and put into a large pot with a lid, and bring to a boil.

- Add the 2 cups of ground up DMT base material and the 1 cup of MAOI material to the boiling water. Hold off on adding the other ingredients until after the initial boiling is complete. Boil with the cover on for at least an hour, stirring occasionally to make sure nothing is burning or sticking to the bottom of the pot.

- After the initial boiling, carefully strain the liquid from the pot and place aside, while keeping the brewing material in the pot.

- Add the remaining 0.5 gallons of water and bring up to a low boil for about 30 minutes with the lid on. Carefully strain this liquid into the first batch of liquid, and either throw away the brewing material, or repeat the flushing process until satisfied you have extracted a majority of the desired products.

- Take the combined liquids and put back into the pot (after brewing material has been removed) and heat up to a simmer. This would be the time to add other teas, herbs, spices, sweeteners, etc., and infuse for 15-20 minutes while stirring as needed.

Depending on what, if any, ingredients you decide to include during this part of the process, you will then have to strain again as/if needed.

You now have a very potent DMT brew in your hands. This liquid can be drunk straight up, it can be used as an ingredient in a cocktail similar to alcohol, it can be added to your coffee or smoothie, it can be frozen in ice cubes for easy portioning, it can be used in cooking to replace water in oatmeal or baked goods, it can be used to dunk your weed brownies in, etc. Once again, a Miracle Molecule!

The next recipe is to make DMT crystals that you smoke or vape. Please note that in this process there are some potentially dangerous materials used, and there is the potential for exploding glass and chemical burns to your skin and eyes. That being said, if you take your time, use the proper precautions, and follow the directions, then the following procedure is straightforward and relatively safe. This is the simple extraction process that I personally use to produce the molecule that helped save my life. As of the writing of this book, I have only used one recipe to make DMT crystals. It is easy and effective. The following is derived from the recipe found on the internet titled "DMT extraction using lye (sodium hydroxide) and naphtha." This page has a disclaimer that states "This guide is provided for informational and educational purposes only. We do not encourage you to break the law and cannot claim any responsibility for your actions." I suggest once again, do not do anything stupid. This recipe would produce what I would call a significant amount of DMT crystals. There are a lot of factors, such as what plant species are used and how many naphtha flushes you decided to do, that will determine the actual yield, but I assure you it will be more than enough for personal use.

The ingredients needed:
- Distilled water
- White vinegar
- Naphtha
- Sodium hydroxide (NaOH), commonly known as lye
- DMT plant base material

The equipment needed:
- Stove or portable cook top
- 2 large pots with lids
- A 2-liter glass jar (or two 1-liter glass jars) with lid(s)
- Large freezer proof glass jar with lid or large Pyrex container with cover for crystallization
- Glass turkey baster
- Freezer
- Chemical resistant gloves (recommended)
- Chemical splash goggles (recommended)

- Respiratory mask rated for noxious gases (recommended)

The extraction process is very simple and uses a traditional acid-based methodology to extract freebase DMT from a liquid solution. In summary, the procedure follows a few basic chemistry steps:

Boil the plant material in the water and vinegar to alter pH. Strain liquid and reduce by evaporation. Mix in lye to alter pH again to make DMT accessible. Add naphtha and shake aggressively to transfer the DMT into solution. Carefully extract the naphtha/DMT solution and allow to reach and stay at freezing point for 48+ hours, which will force the DMT to form crystals and precipitate out. DMT will either attach to the walls of the container or settle to the bottom. Crystals are then transferred to a drying plate and the naphtha is allowed to completely evaporate. What is remaining is freebase DMT in pure form. These crystals can be smoked as is, or turned into vaping cartridges for easy usage.

The most common plants to use for this recipe are *Mimosa hostilis* and *Acacia confusa,* and the root bark is the portion of the plant that is used. It can be purchased as mulch-size chunks, shredded, or in powdered form. The finer the pieces the more surface area is exposed for extraction, and in theory, the more DMT can be pulled from the plant. If you get the larger pieces, you should grind them up in a powerful blender or coffee grinder to maximize the yield. If you get the powder, you will have to filter and strain the liquid to properly separate the solids. I have found the shredded root bark is the best for this recipe, and easiest to use. Freeze and thaw the root bark several times before you begin the recipe; this will cause the cell wall and membrane to break down during a process called lysis, which will allow for higher amounts of DMT to be extracted from the plant material.

Please take proper precautions when handling and mixing the naphtha and lye, and I recommend fully reading the warning labels and information on the packaging of each. Naphtha is a petroleum solvent that is very volatile and is highly flammable. It is harmful if inhaled or swallowed, and should be used only with adequate ventilation. Sodium hydroxide is very hazardous if it comes in contact with your skin or eyes, or if it is ingested or inhaled. Exposure can result in chemical burns and severe damage to skin, eyes, and lungs. Gloves and protective eyewear should be worn when working with lye, and must be added slowly and gradually to the glass jar when mixing to prevent the strong exothermic reaction from cracking the container.

The following recipe is for an extraction using 500 grams of DMT plant base material. Quantities can be scaled up or down as needed, but this amount is an easily manageable volume that provides plenty of product for one's personal use.

1. Combine 1,800 ml of distilled water, 200 ml of white vinegar, and 500 g of DMT plant material into a large pot (A). Cover and bring to a boil on high heat, stirring occasionally to prevent material from burning or sticking to bottom of pot.

2. Reduce heat to medium and cover to maintain a rolling boil. Boil with lid on for at least 1.5 hours, stirring every 5-10 minutes. This gives sufficient time for the DMT to separate from the plant material and be absorbed into the solution, and helps remove any impurities.

3. Strain the solution into another large pot (B), leaving all solids in pot A. There should be approximately 1,000 ml of liquid in pot B.

4. Repeat steps 1 and 2 three more times using fresh water and vinegar each time, reusing the same plant material in pot A each time. This should leave you with approximately 4,000 ml of liquid in pot B.

5. Reduce the contents from pot B from approximately 4,000 ml down to approximately 1,200 ml by boiling without a lid and stirring for as long as needed to properly evaporate off the water and increase the concentration of DMT in the solution.

6. Allow liquid in pot B to cool then pour into 2 L glass jar or evenly into two 1 L glass jars with lids, being careful to keep any settled solids remaining in the pot. Allow this liquid to completely cool to help pre-vent excess heat from the lye reaction from cracking the glass jar. Do not skip this cooling step.

7. Taking proper safety precautions, weigh out 120 g (or 60 g two times if using two jars) of sodium hydroxide. Slowly add in small increments over about 5 minutes. A safe guideline is adding 20 g every 2 minutes and stirring in between. The solution will heat up very rap-idly with the addition of the sodium hydroxide, and it is important to do this step slowly to prevent cracking the glass. The solution will turn grey, then black.

8. The solution should still be warm from the previous step; if not, warm carefully by using a double boil method, or by placing jar in pot and pouring boiling water around it to partially submerge it. Be careful not to put the lid underwater. Solution needs to be warm for DMT extraction to take place. Add 500 ml of naphtha to 2 L jar (or 250 ml to each 1 L jar) and seal tightly. Shake vigorously for several minutes and then let separate for about 10 minutes. Repeat this step 4 or 5 times, keeping the solution warm throughout the process. DMT freebase should now start dissolving into the naphtha.

9. Allow the naphtha layer to fully separate and float to the top. This can take up to several hours; however, if solution is kept warm this process can happen in about an hour. Naphtha layer on top will be completely clear and very distinct from the black sludge below it.

10. Using the glass turkey baster, carefully transfer the naphtha layer into the freezer proof jar or Pyrex container with lid. These containers are where the freebase DMT will crystalize. Make sure you do not transfer any of the black sludge layer. Err on the side of caution during this step to make sure the end product is as pure as possible. The naphtha flushing in step 8 can be repeated several times to get a majority of the DMT out of the solution. I have found that doing 3 flushes with a fresh 500 ml of naphtha will get most of the DMT out. Solution will need to be rewarmed when doing the additional naphtha flushes to allow for separation.

11. Place container in the freezer for at least 48 hours. DMT is insoluble at low temperatures and will gradually crystalize and precipitate out of the naphtha solution.

12. Separate the DMT from the naphtha by slowly pouring off the liquid from the container, making sure to

leave all settled out material behind. A coffee filter can be used for this step; however, I have found this unnecessary if you just take your time. The remaining naphtha can be used in additional flushes.

13. Allow the extracted DMT to fully dry and evaporate all of the naphtha off. This will take several hours and depends on humidity and air flow conditions. Do not try to rush the process by using a fan, the crystals can easily blow away. DMT will dry into a powder-like crystal or a waxy consistency based on the purity.

14. Store in a dry area, in a moisture tight container. Crystals will turn to an oily consistency when heated, but will typically recrystallize when cooled.

CHAPTER 6

DMT Can Help:
Let's Continue the Dialogue

My life-saving exploration and investigation into the Miracle Molecule dimethyltryptamine has given me the confidence to say that we currently have a capable assemblage of intelligent, articulate, and well-intentioned voices spreading the good word about DMT. There is a growing community of respected scientists, prominent social influencers, and intelligent psychonauts that understand DMT can be an integral component in easing mental anguish, unlocking hidden potential, and expanding the collective consciousness of the human species. We must continue to expand the dialogue to ensure that DMT is taken out of the closet and removed from the shelf. We need passionate voices to continue sharing their stories, with the goal of getting DMT into therapeutic tool kits and added back onto the scientific dockets.

Mind expanding chemicals such as DMT have been utilized by our species for thousands and thousands of years on the individual and group level to gain access to ancient wisdom and infinite power, as well as to explore the dimensions of consciousness. Ancient shamans and spiritual leaders understood the beneficial effects of using this natural compound, and gave it the reverence and respect that it deserves. DMT is *not* just another drug to get high off of, it is *not* just some novelty topic for a PhD thesis, and it is *not* just a taboo subject for an aspiring author to discuss in their debut book. DMT allows you to converse with Gods, dance with your guardian Angels, and collaborate with higher beings. DMT has the ability to remove all mental restrictions, obliterate all apprehension, and dissolve physiological boundaries. DMT is the Spirit Molecule, the Miracle Molecule, and in my personal case, the Life-Saving Molecule.

DMT can help. That is undeniable. But the dialogue needs to be continued. There has been some incredible research conducted by scientists like Dr. Terence McKenna, Dr. Dennis McKenna, Dr. Joe Dispenza, Dr. Rick Strassman, and Dr. Steven Barker that is beginning to open our generation's eyes to the potential of this molecule. These are some of the academically trained thinkers who, through their scientific rigor, have helped validate the stories of DMT users by shedding light on the potential and undeniable power this molecule has to alter the human mind, body, and soul. There are contemporary voices like Joe Rogan and Hamilton Morris that help share factual information about personal experiences and future research, and of course there are plenty of psychonauts like myself ready and willing to donate their minds and bodies to the good cause, but much more is needed to properly advance the discussion. We simply need more data.

Speaking from my own personal experience, a large majority of people are uncomfortable talking about DMT, let alone taking it themselves. There are valid reasons to have rational concerns, and DMT is certainly not for everybody, but this natural compound is also not something to be feared or slandered. DMT needs to be studied and understood, not shunned and ignored. The more people exposed to dimethyltryptamine, the more people will appreciate the Miracle Molecule for what it truly is.

One of the biggest obstacles to overcome is DMT's legal status. In most countries it is illegal, and that alone is a huge deterrent for many people. I don't see this changing anytime soon, but there are some reasons to hope that legislation is moving in the right direction in many areas of the world. Positive attitudes towards marijuana and psilocybin mushrooms have been rapidly increasing, and their myriad health benefits are being exposed at a similarly rapid pace.

More and more people are realizing that the normalized and most commonly used mix of prescription pills and alcohol is not the best method for coping with mental and physical ailments. Natural, holistic, and preventive practices are replacing synthetic, conventional, and reactionary medicine. A lot of research has gone into weed and shrooms, and the results are in: they work for a lot of people. The same will be proven with DMT. As more and more doctors and scientists add their names and data in support of future studies, the laws regulating these drugs will hopefully continue to ease and become more reasonable.

It is my personal advice to take some very simple and basic precautions. Don't sell DMT, don't try to profit off of DMT, don't drive with DMT, don't travel with DMT, don't make more DMT than what you personally need, don't share DMT with random people, don't use DMT in public places. My fear of legal repercussions is relatively low because they are directly proportional to my actions and intentions. Don't do stupid shit and you won't get in trouble for doing stupid shit. There will always be some legal liability associated with DMT; however, my experience dealing with law officials is that if you have nothing to hide and are telling the truth, you have little to worry about.

A valid hindrance for many people thinking about using DMT for the first time is the idea of frying your brain, and never being able to return to your normal way of processing life. DMT *will* fry your brain, and you *won't* ever be able to return back to your normal way of processing life. That is the whole point! Keeping with this analogy, DMT will crank up the heat in your brain to allow the congealed blockages to melt away. The increased metaphorical temperature and activity in your brain will provide the conditions needed to synthesize and orchestrate grandiose ideas, as well as lubricate the logistical chain that conveys your thoughts out to the Universal distribution hub. Your brain will certainly get "cooked," and by that I imply zero negative connotations; instead I suggest that your cognitive organ will benefit from DMT's consumption and proper use.

As far as not returning back to your normal way of filtering information, I assure you that you will not want to go back to your chilled, uncooked, doughy brain. It's the equivalent of having a bowl with a glob of cold, raw, uncooked dough versus having a plate with some perfect fried dough, complete with cinnamon and powdered sugar. Your brain will definitely function differently, and you will certainly filter information with a completely new perspective and set of skills.

In my case—as well as those of many other depressed, anxious, or suicidal individuals that I have spoken with on my journey—that is exactly what I needed in order to help make my life enjoyable and full of contentment, as opposed to being angry and overflowing with fear. A new and improved way of interacting with my subconscious thoughts, as well as with my surrounding environment, was just "one toke away" as the late Terrence

McKenna would say. Deciding to take that "one toke" should not be taken lightly, but if the Universe is giving you hints that DMT may be of service to you, it is worth exploring those signs a bit further.

One of the best attributes of DMT is how easily accessible it is to anyone who is seeking it. You don't need to buy it from a shady drug dealer or beg your doctor to write out a prescription. Making your own supply is less complicated, and takes less time than brewing your own beer or growing your own marijuana plants. The monetary cost is nominal, and the amount of DMT that is produced from roughly $100 invested will be enough for quite a few sessions. For the same cost of a fancy latte or craft lager, you can chug a frothy mug of Ayahuasca. For less money than a cheap cigar or nicotine vape cartridge, you can take a puff of the Miracle Molecule. With DMT a very small amount goes a very long way. For most people, a couple hundred dollars' worth of base material will provide enough product to last a full year of personal use. The recipes and procedures that are used to make DMT are extremely simply, are relatively safe, and don't require a lot of time. There is not any complex chemistry involved, nor do you need elaborate or expensive paraphernalia to accomplish the simple extraction. Being in control of the process, from raw material to finished product, also allows you to be 100 percent confident that your DMT is pure and safe.

The biggest obstacle DMT faces on its way to

increased acceptance is the lack of basic information accessible to the general public, combined with the lack of appreciation and recognition by a majority of academic and scientific researchers. I am hoping that in the future, there will continue to be more literature available on DMT, especially considering its potential to help ease many of mankind's most common ailments. There is a stigma and taboo associated with DMT that is unnecessary and extremely unfortunate. We need more calm, educated, and well-spoken proponents. We need more YouTube videos, more podcasts, and more books discussing personal experiences. We need more objective and open-minded studies like the one led by Dr. Strassman, we need more scientists like the McKenna brothers to hand over their analytical minds to the Miracle Molecule, and we need the next generation of profound thinkers to have DMT on the top of their list of worthwhile topics. We need to learn more about the long-term side effects, both negative and positive.

There are far more unanswered questions than agreed upon conclusions. We simply need more data. We need to continue the dialogue. As Dr. Steven Barker stated "...hypotheses have also been offered, suggesting that DMT, as well as other hallucinogens, may provide actual proof of and/or philosophical insights into many of our unanswered questions regarding extraordinary states of consciousness. Regardless of the level and cause of such speculation and hypotheses, it is only scientific research that can inform or refute such thinking. There is no doubt that hallucinogen research has been a forbidden fruit long ripening on the tree of knowledge." The time has come to give dimethyltryptamine the academic attention it deserves so that the general public can get the information they need. Let's pick that "forbidden fruit" and see what that bastard tastes like.

CHAPTER 7

Who the Fuck Are You?

Cʜᴀɴᴄᴇs ᴀʀᴇ ᴛʜᴀᴛ ɪғ ʏᴏᴜ ʜᴀᴠᴇ ᴍᴀᴅᴇ ɪᴛ ᴛʜɪs ғᴀʀ ɪɴ the book, you have either already experienced a DMT session, or are planning to in the near future. So, I must ask: Who the Fuck Are You? Honestly, I want to know *who you are*. What have you learned on your journey, or why do you plan on taking it if you have not yet? Was it what you expected? Was it positive or negative, or a combination of both? Did you have a transformational, life-changing epiphany; or did you simply enjoy some sensory fireworks? How many sessions did you do, and do you plan to continue to use DMT as part of a holistic, well-being lifestyle? Did DMT save your life like it did mine?

As a scientifically trained academic scholar, I feel obligated to assist in data collection. As a philosophically inclined thinker, I am interested in your subjective interpretations. As a psychedelic explorer, I am intrigued in the colorful worlds you may have navigated. As someone who has always felt "alien" on this planet, I am hoping to find my "tribe" and island of misfit DMT psychonauts.

My hope is that with continued data collection from firsthand accounts, the mystique and false information regarding DMT will fade, and the intellectual curiosity and acceptance will increase. I mentioned in the opening chapter how it is *not* my intent to glorify DMT, or push for it to be a mainstream recreational drug. Although I call dimethyltryptamine the "Miracle Molecule," I also respect and appreciate its potential to cause harm, especially if used for nefarious or illegal purposes. My experiences, and those of my friends, have all been extremely positive. We all initially sought out DMT to either help answer a personally challenging question, or to help solve a persistent psychological problem. We all were struggling with mental illness or persistent roadblocks, and we all had lost faith in the traditional medical system to understand our complex and unique issues. We all knew that the solution was not to take a bunch of mind-numbing zombie pills. None of us wanted to run from our problems, we all wanted to bring the fight to them.

Our intention was to be supportive of one another, to share our recipes, to share our DMT, and to share our experiences with a genuine desire to help one another. Not a single dollar was ever exchanged, ever, for any of the DMT sessions we shared. In fact, it is considered an honor and a privilege to donate DMT to someone who needs it. It was with gratitude that we shared our shamanic guidance and expertise. It was with sympathetic and empathetic hearts that we absorbed each other's stories. We all shared the pure and honest desire to *help* our fellow human.

So, I ask once again: Who are you? Are you one of "us"? Are you someone who wants to help move the discussion on DMT in the right direction? Let's continue to add to the DMT community of like-minded, altruistic individuals who can help pull DMT out of obscurity and into the clarifying spotlight. We currently have some great voices and platforms to spread the message. If we reach a critical mass of people, spread enough DMT session stories, the medical and academic communities will have the ammo they need to get the intellectual backing and financial support required to carry out science-based research.

The transformative and spiritual power of DMT that our ancient ancestors utilized can now be proven and documented with brain scans and undeniable physiological changes. There is no doubt that DMT can help alleviate many of our species' mental and physical ailments, but until DMT is further studied, the full potential of dimethyltryptamine will never be realized. As long as the healing powers of the Miracle Molecule are kept as secret, esoteric knowledge accessible only to South American shamans, lab volunteers, or friends of Adam

Butler, we are wasting valuable time and human lives. I will donate my time, I will compile the information, and I will continue to write as many words as needed on the topic of DMT if it will help save just one more life. Please contact me personally with your stories, or if I can help you in any way. I give you my word on discretion and privacy.

My new reality that has manifested from complete destruction, barren ashes, and absolute death, is full of boundless creation, fertile soil, and regenerative life. And I want to share! DMT helped me find my master key, and DMT may help you locate yours. Please be safe, know that you have the power within you to change for the better, and that you are not alone on this journey.

it back up with DMT crystals. Once the crystals are in the cartridge, heat it up with a hairdryer and the crystals will turn into oil. The crystals will start to congeal in cooler temperatures; however, you can easily re-melt as needed using a hairdryer, car heating vents, or (carefully) a lighter. Adding a drop or two of vape pen oil solvent can help prevent congealing backup. Be careful if using a lighter, many cartridges are made of plastic and can melt.

- Try to remove all potential annoyances in the environment that you are about to have your session in. Make sure there are no flies or mosquitoes in the room that will piss you off. Make sure your phone ringer and alarms are off to prevent you from being jarred out of a pleasant train of thought. If you are listening to a wireless speaker, make sure it is fully charged. The last thing you want to hear seven minutes and twenty-two seconds into a meditative trance track is "BATTERY LOW" in the voice of your least favorite middle school teacher—that or a spam phone call about your utility bill.

- Don't freak out if your DMT crystals turn into DMT wax. Higher temperatures and higher humidity can and will change the consistency. In my experience, this does not alter the strength of the DMT, and does not really change how you smoke/vape it.

- Ayahuasca can sneak back up on you after you think the journey is over. I drank a pretty large dose one evening, and had a wonderful four- to five-hour session on the beach. I then went to sleep thinking I had completed most of my trip. I woke up about two hours later in complete pandemonium and chaos. I woke up in the middle of a mental mind fuck! It took me a moment to realize where I was, and what the hell was happening. It was not that I had a "bad" experience; it was more like I was waking up after being thrown from a plane and was in freefall. After the initial shock of seeing the ground coming at me at the speed of gravity, I could reach back and open my parachute and compose myself.

- Have a pen and paper ready to record your journey. Keeping a journal to record your sessions is a great way to document your DMT induced self-actualization. There will be words and phrases that keep being repeated in your head when you are in the deepest depths of a DMT session; I suggest writing them down for further reflection, and integration into your life. Three-word phrases repeated three times was something that seemed to happen often with myself and friends as we were coming out of the DMT session. "I love you, I love you, I love you"; "Let it go, let it go, let it go"; "Down the middle, down the middle, down the middle"; "It just is, it just is, it just is," are some examples.

- Taking a hot shower and/or bath is highly enjoyable shortly after smoking DMT. Use some common sense here to prevent slipping on a wet floor or getting your pipe/pen wet, but done properly, this can be a very relaxing experience. This is probably best done with a partner for added protection (and potential pleasure).

- Being overwhelmed with emotion and crying is very common as you come out of a DMT session. Be very careful about blowing your nose too hard. I made a slightly aggressive blow into a tissue, and the following sensation in my sinus area was not pleasant.

- Stare into a campfire or fireplace to relax and contemplate life while on DMT. Your efforts will be worth your time.

- Don't assume everyone will be "cool" with you using DMT, or talking about it. Not everyone will be.

CHAPTER 9

Public Announcement:
Love Thy Neighbor

My painful experience with mental depression and having suicidal thoughts ultimately transformed my understanding of the importance of human-to-human interaction, and the power of sharing love. In my year or so of traveling the country, I drove from Rhode Island to California twice, visited Kansas City (Missouri, not Kansas—don't confuse the two) like eight times, stopped at most major cities on my way from Maine to Miami, hung out in the Cascade Mountains, Rocky Mountains, and the Blue Ridge Mountains, lived on the beach in northern California for two weeks, spent days roaming the streets of Las Vegas, meditated in Mexico for over a week, and slept in an ice hotel in Canada, to name a few places.

Along my travels I had intimate and personal conversations with people who lived in the city, the country, the swamps, the mountains, and the desert. I shared hugs and tears with young women, old men, several cats and dogs, as well as a bunch of trees. I heard stories of success and goals achieved, as well as tales of devastation and crushed dreams. I had dinner with millionaires overlooking the Pacific Ocean at luxury restaurants, as well as shared joints with homeless wanderers in piss-filled streets. Every individual that I had the good fortune to interact with all had the same basic need and desire to be appreciated as a unique individual, listened to, respected, and loved. This sounds so basic, but the majority of people today do not even know how to appreciate, listen to, respect, and love themselves, let alone their neighbors. Once I experienced what the power of love did for my own psyche and well-being, I knew I would spend the rest of my life trying to help as many people as I could, break the cycle of self-hatred and hatred of others, by simply showing them the power of love.

My year-long spiritual journey and personal sabbatical began full of hate, anger, and despair; it ended overflowing with love, joy, and hope. I shared my pain, flaws, and rawness with random strangers, and in return they comforted me with stories of their own struggles and life challenges. Over time I realized how important the companionship, help, and love of other humans was to my own self recovery. By drawing strength from the people around me, I was able to get my life back in order; by sharing my tears, hugs, and empathy with others, I was able to continue the cycle.

I used to shy away from both giving and receiving love due to pain associated with past traumas. I now try to share love with everyone I cross paths with. Martin Luther King Jr. stated "Darkness cannot drive out darkness; only light can do that. Hate cannot drive out hate; only love can do that." I used to wallow in darkness and hate, and now I frolic in light and love. Please do your part to love thy neighbor, you never know when you will be that neighbor that needs love.

With Love,
Adam Butler

A Call to Action

THANK YOU FOR TAKING THE TIME TO READ THIS BOOK. I hope its contents have provided a small amount of helpful information and insight into the Miracle Molecule DMT. If DMT has piqued your interest, I suggest looking into the work of the scientists and influencers mentioned within these pages to educate and inspire you with their research and stories. There is a psychedelic movement picking up steam, and it is reflected in the countless PhD professors, programs, and students that are doing amazing work and sharing their data and conclusions through their publications and conferences. My experience reaching out and listening to this community is that they are extremely gracious in giving personal time with their responses, and are excited and willing to share their expertise. I recommend following these universities, research labs, and individuals on their social media platforms or newsletters, as well as reaching out to them if you have any specific questions.

If you have any questions or comments for me directly, or would like to share your story about your

DMT experiences, please feel free to email me at BooksbyAdamButler@gmail.com I promise discretion, integrity, and honesty in my collection and response to any emails I may receive. If you would like to support the success and spread of my message, please take a moment to give a review if you purchased from an online store or have the e-book.

If you know a friend or family member who may benefit from the information in this book, please give them this copy to borrow, or get them one as a gift. Once the dialogue has begun, the healing process can begin, and a relevant book is a great conversation starter. The heartfelt discussions I have had about DMT with my friends, how it has helped us deal with our depression and unique mental illness issues; these talks have been life changing and lifesaving for all of us. If you see someone you love who is in a dark place, please help them bring some light back to their life anyway you can, even just by giving them a sincere hug.

Alicia's Angle

I'T'S IMPORTANT THAT THE AUTHOR'S STATEMENTS ON sublime sex be substantiated, and it is with great pleasure and purpose that I impart my perspective. As Adam's spirited partner on multiple levels, I can confirm that our shared psychedelic experiences, with DMT specifically, have led to earth-shattering energy exchanges—multiple orgasms aside. And as an occupational therapist, mother, and woman coming from high childhood adversity, my viewpoint on the power of DMT is all the more relevant.

Transcendent Sex as Soul Dialysis

I treasure the depths of connection a shared DMT experience can create between companions. It's amazing how enjoying your lover deep inside of you can also bring a deeper understanding of yourself, and the core of your relationships. While fitting bodies together like puzzles pieces, you're noticing how *everything* fits in conjunction with each other in this world and in others. The filling, the in, out, back, forth, sucking, pushing, syncopated breathing, contracting and releasing. Letting bodily fluids go and simultaneously letting so much pain go. And relishing in the revelation that the acknowledgement of that pain can somehow bring such anchoring euphoria. Co-regulation through plaque removing penetration! And as the plaque removal process takes place, you become more open to giving and receiving. Not only in regards to orgasms and self-love, but to a transformative equanimity found through feeling a new relationship with your fears, while not feeling alone.

Having transcendental sex to this degree seems to create a sort of vortex, or circling, that is a figure 8, that is endless, that takes the erotic bliss of pleasure and electricity between partners and opens a door to your own nervous system regulation. Coursing between you is not just cum, but a spiritual soup felt between nucleotides. I have witnessed the rehabilitative recalibrations that can occur from rinsing and repeating with this miracle molecule. By virtue of surrendering, syncing and sinking into intimacy with someone special and safe, I have found inner realms open and abounding. The doors of possibility seem endless and unlocked for reclamation of self. Leading to the life-changing realization that YOU are the open door that you have been searching for. A door that's always been open.

Finding adequate words to capture the essence of transcendental sex is a beautiful challenge, as there can be such poetry in locking into one another, that is only amplified during a psychedelic experience. Coital circling surpasses energy dances at some point and somehow becomes a music that you can see and manipulate. During DMT sessions, sounds seem so expansive, and you sink into the symphony as some sort of savant conductor, effortlessly highlighting the different instruments in your environment, and attuning to your own vibrations in an eye-opening way with each breath, squeal, moan, word. Therein, on DMT (which then ends up permeating life in this dimension too), the repetitive nature of our words and how subconscious and rhythmically responsive they can become—for the good—makes you realize the impact of negative self-talk and disconnected automatic replies. It can be of serious detriment to stay stuck within those typically trauma-driven cycles, like letting the scratched CD stay where it is skipping (which keeps highlighting the scratch and not the rest of the album). Exploring DMT on your own or with a conscious companion then becomes a chance to fill in those scratches and play the music, feel the music, be the music. As the conductor (ME?!) leads a duet between the crickets and the humming fan, loving words escape so knowingly, they become little mantras that are part of this engaging concert of connected vibrations. But to say them and repeat them inside of the music that you are making through making love was, and is astounding. I'm saying them to myself and I'm hearing them at a deeper level, in a realm that feels more truthful, more real. To me, this captures what Alan Watts stated as, 'music beyond belief,' and that is so fucking therapeutic—because that music is love beyond our limiting beliefs!

Therapeutic Potential

I have long been a proponent of mindful, creative journaling for processing thoughts. I see the value of its expressive ventilation onto paper, and how it gives clarity to what's in your head. Prior to psychedelic use, writing was already a personal practice used for self-reflection, as I appreciate the emotional malleability and non-identification it can allow. A DMT experience, however, is unlike any reflective journal prompt. It is like opening up the book of yourself, getting a peek behind the pages, deep into the inner gears of a publishing company, where you are illuminating the manuscript, and rewriting chapters. It is where you are authenticating your authorship in this wild ass create-your-own-magic-musings-and-misadventures book, italicizing your own truths, identifying and editing imposter syndrome and trauma, heartbreak and hard lessons without minimization, disassociation or disconnection. Each time this 'book' closes, I have affirmed again and again the truth behind how connected I can be to myself and to the Universe. Entering DMT space with the intent of self-exploration and healing can allow admittance to a powerful awareness, with reminders of how accessible this can be even by 'simply' reclaiming our breathing and remembering our own light.

Needless to say, the use of psychedelics in my own intimate practices has strengthened my connection to self, and this has permeated into all aspects of my life. Then to consider DMT use through my clinical lens, I can zoom out with clarity on the populations that could be positively impacted with its use. Through the powerful prismatic microscope of DMT and my occupation helping patients reform meaning in their lives, I can see how large-scale fostering of openness and connection could rewrite collective consciousness in a world-changing way. As a society, psychedelics offer an incredible and urgent chance to address mental health in general, through expanding willingness to reframe fears and approach relating differently. How much better could our world be, both in and out of the bedroom?

Having personally experienced the retained benefits on my own mental health, and having provided intervention for illness and trauma across the lifespan as an occupational therapist, I see how grave and necessary the use of this potent psychoactive substance can be as a medicine. We are all in our own ways, covered in plaque from systemic injustices, self-abandonment, sedentary lifestyle, attachment insecurities, nutritional deficiencies and financial challenges. Undoubtedly, the pandemic, skin hunger, and associated isolation only further compacts this plaque over time, ultimately keeping us sick. This stress on the mind and body can instigate inflammation which leads to stroke, dementia, insidious artery clogging, heart attack and systemic issues like rheumatoid arthritis and cancer. Not to mention their correlation with sexual and intimacy issues, which further depletes important neurotransmitters. Thus, the tie to mental/physical wellness is undeniable, with any additional stress further perpetuating the high cost of healthcare and increased suicide rates. Living with that health-related heaviness on low social supports, and with low self-worth can lead to feeling like the only option is long-term therapy and years of paying for medication with side effects that can be very disruptive to quality of life. These external manifestations have cellularly-associated changes that correspond with abundant evidence of cognitive and psychological ramifications of chronic stress. There is a growing body of information on the neurochemical action of how DMT, which based on the receptor site activation shown in studies, is both physiologically rewiring long-term potentiated synapses, and in turn spiritually changing tracks to reroute the 'train' of your brain. DMT could be the medicine many of us living with mental health challenges today need, and offers a solution that could shorten both cost and length of treatment, while allowing more humans to lead purposeful, pleasureful lives.

Message from Shaman Shawn

"EVERY DAY OF MY EARTHLY LIFE IT BECAME MORE apparent that the architects of our society claim something is 'Bad' when it is inherently 'Good,' and in the next breath they try to convince us that their systems of control and oppression are for our own good... and they have the majority of us fooled into believing these lies. With just a few breaths of smoke from a plant that the Creator put on this planet for us to use and benefit from, all of those lies are wiped away like mud off the windshield of our existence. Then you can see that God is real and loves us all absolutely! Fear not earthly death my friends, it is neither the beginning nor the end, and take time to appreciate every moment we have here together in this beautiful space."

Shaman Shawn

About the Author

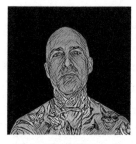

Adam Butler is a psychedelic philosopher and passionate DMT psychonaut focusing on mental health, neuroplasticity, self-exploration, and the extreme limits of human potential and ability. Combining an academically trained intellect, empathetic heart, and life-hardening experiences, Adam has found his niche in helping others overcome the fear associated with PTSD, depression, sexual repression, and addiction. By incorporating psychedelic compounds with deep meditation, lucid dreaming, and tantric practices he has changed from being an over worked, over-weight, stressed-out alcoholic asshole into a balanced, healthy, and sober friend and mentor to many.

Made in the USA
Middletown, DE
16 June 2023

32750798R00056